Pray 'Bout It, Girl

JILLIAN ROUSE

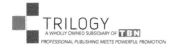

Pray 'Bout It Girl

Trilogy Christian Publishers
A Wholly Owned Subsidary of Trinity Broadcasting Network
2442 Michelle DriveTustin, CA 92780
Copyright © 2023 by Jillian Rouse

For information, address Trilogy Christian Publishing
Rights Department, 2442 Michelle Drive, Tustin, CA 92780.
Trilogy Christian Publishing/ TBN and colophon are trademarks of Trinity Broadcasting Network.
For information about special discounts for bulk purchases, please contact Trilogy Christian Publishing.

10 9 8 7 6 5 4 3 2 1

Library of Congress Cataloging-in-Publication Data is available.

ISBN 979-9-89041-635-3

ISBN (ebook) 979-9-89041-636-0

Dedication

To my mom, Dina Kimbrough, a.k.a. DinaKim, who never stopped believing in me and pushing me, even when she didn't fully understand. Thank you for shining a light on my darkness and helping me refocus and readjust. Thank you for answering the phone in the middle of the night to nothing but sorrow and hurt, and being strong enough to encourage me through the pain. I thank God for creating you for the purpose of being my mother; there's no other I'd want.

Thank you for helping me battle my bipolar disorder alongside Jesus!

I love you.

Preface

My Story

Hey, girl! My name is Jillian, and I created this journal with the intention of helping other Christian (no matter where you are) women get closer to God and also address any mental health issues or concerns.

In November 2014, I entered into ministry at the age of 20. I wasn't ready, and I fell back into the world and fell victim to my flesh. Throughout the time that has passed, I heard God speaking to me, telling me to get back on track, get into the Word, and continue my walk with Jesus.

During the time that I fell off track, my mental health worsened. I attempted suicide three times and also had been admitted to a psych ward. I was diagnosed with Bipolar II disorder. I became deathly depressed and couldn't find a way out. My hypomania led me into a world of extreme debt and bad choices.

After I left my place at Jesus' feet, my life turned into a pit of darkness. Of course I had good moments, like marrying my husband, finding some purpose in job choices, and creating a mental health journal (*My Hidden Jewels*) but overall, I suffered.

In 2022, yes, eight years later, I rededicated my life to God and vowed to live in His vision and purpose for my life: ministry, mental health, physical health, and wealth. I was ordained as a minister in April 2023.

Do I still have struggles and bad days? Of course, but the load has been lightened since giving my life back to God; He's helping me carry my troubles.

With this journal, I hope you start or continue following God's direction, His plan for your life, and can focus on Him and also your mental health.

May healing, peace, and joy be with you. God is with you, ALWAYS!

Introduction

Sometimes in your walk with Christ, you'll feel like He's left your side. Sometimes in your journey through mental health/illness, you'll feel that He's completely abandoned you. But I'm here to tell you, those are the times He's the closest. I've experienced this for myself.

"Do not be afraid or discouraged, for the Lord will personally go ahead of you. He will be with you; he will neither fail you nor abandon you." (Deuteronomy 31:8 NLT)

Every thought heard, tear wiped, and promise kept. That's the reason I'm alive today, because He was there and He kept me.

This Christian mental health prayer journal was designed to help you rekindle your relationship with God, bring Him back into your life, and show you that He has not forgotten you or your name.

Take your time with this journal; it shouldn't be completed in one day. Perfect relationships take time; perfect your relationship with God, take your time.

Date started ___January___ ___23___ 20_24___
(The date you decided to "Pray 'Bout It, Girl")

Order of Service

(JUST LIKE CHURCH)

Dear Heavenly Father,

I come here on this specific page to first thank You for allowing this woman to pick up this journal and wanting to better her relationship with You and herself. I want to ask for You to protect her through this season, provide her with focus to complete this front to back, and for her to be open and honest with herself and You. I pray for peace in any situation that has a strong hold on her. I pray that she be more like You at the end of this journey. I pray that distractions be taken away, that she takes her time but doesn't forget about it, either. I'm asking for an increase not only in her faith and walk and calling with You, but also for an increase in her confidence in her ability to carry and live it out. I pray that she become the woman You've created, and she'll begin to walk boldly in that.

These things I ask in Your Son Jesus' name,

Amen

Being a Woman

Being a woman is hard, and let nobody tell you it isn't, so let us chat about that briefly.

We have so much that goes on within our lives. First of all, we have monthly cycles, and if you're like me they are pretty bad. Next, some of us have husbands and have to live up to their standards and ours within the marriage. If you're lucky, you'll be blessed with a husband like mine, who makes married life pretty great. Lastly, some women are blessed with children. (Although I haven't been yet, I have pups for the time being.) Dealing with such fragile individuals and all their needs has to be a challenge and mental strain at times. Of course you love your children, but I can imagine it can be stressful.

Women have been silenced too long and sometimes that still affects us, in all aspects of life. Sometimes we feel defeated even before the battle begins, and that's just sad. Luckily, I know someone who looks at us like diamonds and rubies, and treats us no different than our brothers.

Being a woman can also be hard due to depression. Did you know that there are different types? Depression affects women more than men, although men take their lives more often than women due to more lethal methods. Women are often more depressed.

WOMEN ARE TURNING IT AROUND!

If you're feeling like life is too hard, or even if life isn't for you, please know that it is. You were created for a purpose, and I'm not just saying that; I really mean it. You were created for a purpose that may be even bigger than your vision for your life. God makes no mistakes.

Even if you just help one other person with your testimony, one other sister, brother, friend, or even stranger, that's all that matters, right?

There are so many strong women in the Bible. Let's name a few:

Deborah- Prophetess
Esther- A Queen
Even EVE- The first woman created

Even though Eve disobeyed God, she has the ability to teach us a lesson, to show us what full submission should be, and what being disobedient can do. Disobedience can cause generational curses. She teaches us the importance of self-control and ignoring our flesh.

So yeah, we're out here seeking help from counselors and psychiatrists, but also staying prayed up and in our Word, I'm proud of every single woman taking control of her life, even the smallest portion. Life is hard; being a woman has its challenges, but God has a purpose for your life, a purpose more divine than imagined.

Let's get to it!

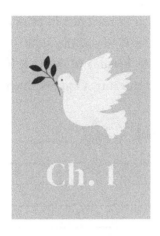

Safe Place

"He who dwells in the secret place of the Most High shall
abide under the shadow of the Almighty. I will say of the Lord,
" He is my refuge and my fortress; My God, in Him I will trust.""

(Psalms 91:1-2 NKJV)

How this speaks to me:

With and in the Lord, our God, is a safe place where we can
live and not be afraid. Trusting in God brings me peace and an
understanding that with Him, I cannot be alone, afraid, or truly die.
Dwelling in the secret place is sacred and those who dwell within are
safe under His shadow or care.

Know that God loves you, even when you feel unknown, forgotten,
or unlovable. I mean, He gave His only Son to free us from our sins.

Feeling safe in His arms is important, and trusting Him and all
He has for your life is the first step. God wants the best version of

you, who He created you to be. Trust in Him and follow His voice; you're safe when you have God on your side!

Tip: Girl, you're safe, loved, and wanted! If no one else tells you that, I am, and more importantly God continually is!

How does this speak to you? _____

_____

_____

_____

_____

_____

_____

_____

_____

_____

_____

_____

_____

_____

_____

_____

_____

_____

_____

_____

_____

_____

_____

_____

PRAYER

Dear Heavenly Father,

I pray for the woman using this journal for her healing journey and for her walk with You. I pray that You will meet her where she's at, wrap Your arms around her, and continue to walk with her. She needs You now more than ever before. The world can be so cold sometimes, judgments, stigmas, hatred, and so on. I pray you protect her from harsh words. I pray that she moves along in this journal with patience and confidence, that each time she reads a word or writes one herself, she is changed. Little by little, she'll change. And I pray You help her to become whole in every area needed. In Jesus' name we pray,

Amen

Jesus

Jesus and His love is so amazing to me, I can't even explain it all of the way. There are countless times where I've felt His love, warmth, embrace, acceptance, and protection. Even when I fell off and "back" (happened more than once) into the world, I still felt it. (I think a lot of my protection from being in the world came from my praying grandparents and mother).

When I think of the goodness of Jesus, and ALL He's done for me, I can't do anything except cry. You know how some people cut a step, and some are blessed to speak in tongues, my praise is tears. Every Sunday I grab tissues on the way to my seat and when I get home after service I throw away the wet tissues from my purse or coat pocket.

There are so many times when I should have been dead. And I know every Christian says that, but it's really true! I've had my fair share of dangerous situations, abusive relationships, suicide attempts, and a lot of dumb teenage decisions; and yet I'm here alive to testify and tell my story.

Even in my mistakes I've always been welcomed back, to a safe place, a place free from my mistakes, drama, sins, or even my mind. (My anxiety can be powerful) A place where I don't have to explain myself, be questioned, or be judged. A place I'm forgiven and told to push on.

RELATIONSHIP BUILDING WITH GOD

Over the next few pages, you'll answer questions, search the Bible, and start to build your own relationship with our Lord and Savior.

The importance of Jesus, what is it?

_____

_____

_____

Have you been giving your all to God recently?

Yes or No

Why or why not?

_____

_____

_____

What's your "forever" verse?

Why does this match your life? Why is it so important?

_____

_____

_____

What is one way He has turned your weakness into strength?

_____

_____

_____

Find a Psalm you love and write it here.

_____

_____

_____

Why did you select this specific Psalm?

_____

_____

_____

What's your favorite way to spend time with God?

_____

_____

_____

What song has been stuck in your head this week? What does it mean for your life in this current season?

_____

_____

_____

The purpose of the previous activity is to start or continue your relationship with Christ. Now let's dive into your spiritual healing.

A Safe Place with Jesus Christ

What is a safe place to you? What does it look and feel like? What about knowing God loves you makes you feel safe? Who on Earth makes you feel the safest?

1. _____

2. _____

3. _____

What are some safe places you can go to if in trouble? (mentally, spiritually, physically)

1. _____
2. _____
3. _____

If you could talk to your younger self and keep her safer and prepare her more for the world, what would you say?

What can you do to protect your safe place within yourself?

1. _____
2. _____
3. _____
4. _____
5. _____

What should you do to protect your safe place with God and why should that be a priority?

_____
_____
_____
_____
_____
_____
_____
_____
_____
_____
_____

_____

_____

_____

_____

_____

_____

_____

_____

_____

"I Shall Not Fear for I Know the Lord!"

There's nothing to fear when you're walking alongside the Lord. I know it can be hard to see that sometimes, but having faith in God and His power will remove any doubts you have and help to increase your faith.

Ever been scared to ride a plane or ride in someone else's car? Did that cause you to pray? Obviously, you survived.

Next time you flew or rode in that person's car, did you feel better? More confident? More protected?

Of course, we still pray for protection in all that we do, but we have fewer doubts and more faith.

Jesus and a Psychiatrist

Let me be the first to say it: "You can have Jesus and see a psychiatrist!"

There's nothing wrong with that, as long as your faith and trust ultimately is in God.

God had (has) a purpose for doctors, lawyers, teachers, and preachers, let us not forget.

Sometimes, some people will need medication in order to help them live the life God gave them. Jesus can heal any man (or woman) but sometimes, in the meantime, while we wait for our miracle, we need help!

Being in counseling can be a safe place. They are bound by HIPPA laws. There's nothing like talking to God, but talking to another person be a starting point.

I started seeing a psychiatrist in 2020 after having recurrent suicidal ideations. One day at work, I called my mom crying, begging her to take me to the hospital. See, I've been working in mental health for over five years so I know "all the signs and symptoms of mental health":

Let's see... Depression isn't always sad and locked up in the house; depression can be a person faking a smile, going to work, graduating college, and so on. Depression can look different in everyone. Anxiety is the feeling of excessive worrying. Everyone has anxiety at some point, but the number of episodes, duration, and intensity is what makes anxiety normal or an illness. Just to speak on two mental illnesses.

I started having mental health issues around the age of 12 but it really intensified when I was 15, in high school. So I basically went 12 years with no help from a doctor and I wasn't in my Word or speaking about it to my family, so no one was praying for that specifically. We didn't even know what "it" was. By 2014 I already had two suicide attempts.

In 2020, I was diagnosed with bipolar II disorder by two doctors (psychiatrists). I felt even more hopeless and helpless. Now I had a title to my pain, a title with so much stigma.

I carried that weight hard. After my psych ward stay, my mom and grandfather (Rev. Clifford Kimbrough) intensified their prayers. I started attending my current church and my pastor (Mark T. Jackson) prayed for me (at least) every Sunday. With all those prayers, tears, and cries, the weight started to shift. And now I'm writing this guided journal, to help the next girl find God in the midst of a mess and pain, and remind you to still praise Him even when it's hard.

Tip: Pray always, but speak to your spiritual leader along with your mental health provider. Having both on board, together, will help aid in your healing process. Having multiple supports will also aid in your healing process, not feeling so alone. It can also help by allowing you to distribute the weight of your pain and problems, having multiple people to help you cope, learn, and grow.

Are you currently in counseling (spiritual and/or mental)?

Yes or No

What are three things you need to get off of your chest and receive help for?

1. _____
2. _____
3. _____

What are three goals you can work on in counseling?

1. _____
2. _____
3. _____

How would working through these issues and reaching your goals help you get closer to God through counseling?

Traumas, Pain, and Hurt

Write about those things listed above; this is a private journal so let it all out. Releasing the pain is the first step to begin healing, growing, and becoming resilient.

_____
_____
_____
_____
_____
_____
_____

_____

_____

_____

_____

_____

_____

_____

_____

_____

_____

_____

_____

_____

LOVE, HOPE, AND HEALING

Now that you have had time to reopen unhealed wounds, cry, and shed some unbearable emotions, let's heal the correct way, together.

If you ever told someone your situation, who believed you?

_____

_____

_____

How did that make you feel?

_____

_____

_____

If you never told anyone, why not?

_____

_____

_____

"I forgive myself for..."

_____

_____

_____

"I forgive _____

for..." _____

_____

_____

What makes you feel complete and whole? Anything positive.

_____

_____

_____

When do you feel the most like yourself?

_____

_____

_____

I love myself the most when...

_____

_____

_____

What are some healthy coping skills you can use to get through this?

_____

_____

_____

How can you challenge yourself to get through this?

_____

_____

_____

A Prayer for Today

Dear God,

Thank You for... _____

_____

_____

_____

Please (ask for what you need and want)... _____

_____

_____

_____

I'm sorry for (confess and ask forgiveness)... _____

_____

_____

_____

Protect me from... _____

_____

_____

_____

In Jesus' name,

Amen

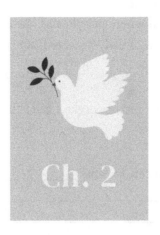

The Past is Not My Future

"Whom God hath set forth to be a propitiation through faith in his blood, to declare his righteousness for the remission of sins that are past, through the forbearance of God."

(Romans 3:25 KJV)

How this speaks to me:

Because of the sacrifice of God's son, Jesus, we do not have to live in our past. We can make mistakes and be forgiven all because Jesus has died for our sins. Having faith in Jesus and trusting in the Word sets us free, our past and past mistakes cannot hold nor bind us.

The past is simply that, the past. When we declare and act as new people in Christ within the world, no mistake or sin can be said to make us who we are.

We live in a world where people and ourselves are our toughest critics, where God has already accepted our apology and made us white as snow.

Tip: Your past isn't picture perfect, but it'll make a great story of how you made it over.

How does this speak to you? _____

_____

_____

_____

_____

_____

_____

_____

_____

_____

_____

_____

_____

_____

_____

_____

_____

_____

_____

_____

_____

_____

PRAYER

Lord, we come to You as humbly as we know how, asking You in this chapter of this book and season of this woman's life, that you cover her but also let her know it's okay. Her past is not her future, and all sins can be forgiven. All hurt can be healed. Let Your Holy Spirit move into her heart and guide her and comfort her. Please let her know that you are Alpha and Omega, the beginning and the end; without You there is no other. Let her know that no matter what physical or mental struggles she faces, that You ultimately have the final say. We may not always understand, but the plan is divine. Lastly, I ask for You to drive her out of a dark place; show her a glimpse of light so she knows there is hope. Bless anyone in her life that's giving diagnosis and aftercare. These things we ask in Jesus' name,

Amen

He Heals

Girl, listen, I've prayed and asked God for healing for so many things (for myself, my mind, my body, my friends and family). And I've witnessed healing in those areas. Its miraculous! I've seen women conceive that doctors said never would. I've met a girl who basically died and came back to life. And there's me, no longer living with a black raincloud over her head all the time, so deep down dark that life didn't seem like an option.

Pray this prayer with me. And pray for your healing.

"Precious Father, I come humbly before You to first thank You for all You've protected me from and healed me from in the past. I need Your healing once again. I'm sick in some way (add what you need to be healed from) and I kneel before You, hands stretched out to touch the hem of Your garment, with even that I'll be healed. Lord, I need to be healed from my past hurts, traumas, and pain, so I'm reaching out to You to receive healing, so I may be made new.

These things we ask in Jesus' name,

Amen

How has Jesus healed you in the past?

_____

_____

_____

What miracles have you seen Him do (big or small)?

_____

_____

_____

Take a second and thank Him for all He's done for you!
(Write your praise here)_____

_____

_____

_____

What have you seen, firsthand, God do in another person's life that healed them?

_____

_____

_____

"And he said unto her, Daughter, thy faith hath made thee whole, go in peace, and be whole of thy plague."

(Mark 5:34 KJV)

What story about healing in the Bible resonates with you the most? Why?

_____

_____

_____

Scriptures:

_____

_____

_____

_____

_____

_____

_____

_____

Girl, I know,

Sometimes, it is just too hard to talk about the things we are ashamed of within our lives (bad relationships, financial issues, addictions, sexual assaults, etc.). The issues then become a burden in our hearts, they become heavy and too difficult to deal with on a daily basis. The burdens feel just as that, and we don't want to burden anyone else with them or we just feel outright disgusted with ourselves for allowing it to happen or getting that bad. We don't want to be judged or belittled, either.

Oftentimes we don't seek out therapy because we don't want to share our story, pain, and embarrassments with a stranger who may or may not understand. The insane part is, we don't have to tell somebody new, somebody who won't understand; we can talk to Jesus about it.

Psalm 147: 3 (KJV) reads, "He health the broken in heart, and bindeth up their wounds.

I mean, if that's not confirmation that you can and shall be healed from those dark places, I don't know what is.

Don't sit in your pain; pray to God and ask to be healed!

"Lord, I'm hurting, please heal me."
It can be as simple of a prayer as that!

Here you'll jot down healing you're asking for yourself and others. Do it however you like! Write it, pray over it, and cross it out when it happens... Write it, pray over it, and check it ✓ when it's done... However you like; you have room, just make sure you pray over each entry, continuously. I'll start it off for you.

Sound mental health for myself and every woman in the world.

PRAY 'BOUT IT GIRL

_____

_____

_____

_____

_____

_____

_____

_____

_____

_____

_____

_____

_____

_____

_____

_____

_____

_____

_____

_____

_____

_____

"JESUS CAN HEAL THE THINGS

YOU WON'T TALK ABOUT."

Helping Me to Heal

As stated previously, oftentimes we don't seek out help from professionals like therapists because it can be hard to trust and open up to a complete stranger. "And what if I don't like them?"

All are valid points.

But what if you really like them, they help you tremendously, and they even help you in your journey in getting closer to God unintentionally? (Intentionally, if you have a Christian counselor.)

My therapist has done just that in two years' time. Before her, I had multiple therapists I did not really click with and I'd stop going. It would be months and I'd fall into a dark place again and I'd need to find someone new.

When I met my current therapist, I was like, "Here we go again. I'll share my story and get a little advice, and after three sessions I'll realize I don't really care for her. LIKE ALWAYS."

But I gave her a chance, and with her I've learned so much about myself and the effect I have on my own life and others, that I've had to check myself, my attitude, and even my spirit. This unintentionally has brought me closer to God.

I'm a Girl Who...

Loves_____

Wants to_____

Is doing it for_____

Believes in_____

Will one day_____

Is sorry for_____

Deserves_____

Is looking for_____

Needs_____

Wants_____

Is deciding to_____

Is interested in_____

Desires_____

What are Positive Affirmations?

I recently went to a girls' confidence brunch and the host asked the question stated above... little girls 4-13 gave their best definition. I heard things like, "Positive affirmations are things that make you feel better about yourself" and other similar renditions. It was a beautiful sight to see, these young girls learning and speaking on such an underrated topic, one in which I struggle with in my adult life, remembering to chant over and over to myself in order to boost my self-esteem and confidence.

The girls were also asked to name an affirmation and remember to say it at least once a day.

As hard as it seems, it's really simple. It's setting an alarm on your phone or putting a sticky note somewhere you go every day, like above your bathroom sink.

It's important to remind ourselves that WE MATTER and WE ARE STRONG and WORTHY. Sometimes in the shuffle of life, we forget. It's our responsibility to remind ourselves. If we don't, who will?

"I AM A CHILD OF THE KING."

Positive Affirmations

I am safe.
I am loved.
It's not my fault what happened to .
I am worthy.
I deserve good things.
I am human
I am healing and becoming the person I was designed to be.

Now, create your own!

1_____

2_____

3_____

4_____

5_____

POSITIVE SELF TALK

Changing from Negative to Positive

What have you said negatively about yourself or your abilities and how can you change it?

Negative Thought	Rewired Thought
This is too hard	This will take effort and time

_____

_____

_____

_____

_____

_____

Why this is important: we can be our toughest critics. The things we tell ourselves we often believe, because it's us! Rewiring our thoughts and battling negative thoughts with positive thoughts will help us defeat our minds and insecurities. This will then allow us to be more confident and believe in ourselves more.

Tip: Write the things you want to tell your negative thoughts on sticky notes and place them all around the house, at your job, or even in your car. Seeing and repeating these positive affirmations/thoughts will help rewire your brain.

Unresolved Grief

Denial, Anger, Bargaining, Depression, Acceptance

Girl, did you know grief could be caused by anything you lose? The loss of a person, of course, but also the loss of an addiction, car, or even an animal. Everyone grieves differently, too! I like to use 9/11 as an example. Some people returned to work as soon as it resumed, some took months off, and some never returned due to the PTSD they were assumed to have had.

What is your grief you're currently dealing with?

_____

_____

_____

How are you currently coping (negative and positive)?

_____

_____

_____

How should you really be coping with it? List some healthy coping skills.

_____

_____

_____

Who can you talk to in order to feel better? _____

_____

_____

_____

Finish the Sentence- Grief

_____

_____

_____

Right now you feel...

_____

_____

_____

The grief is the hardest when...

_____

_____

_____

The thing/feeling you'll miss the most about is

_____

_____

_____

Things have been different since the loss by...

_____

_____

_____

Have you had any regrets regarding the loss?

_____

_____

_____

How has this loss impacted you the most?

_____

_____

_____

Would you like to say goodbye, one last time?

Yes or No

Goodbye Letter

Date: _____

To: _____

I am saying goodbye because...

_____
_____
_____

I remember when...

_____
_____
_____

You taught me...

_____
_____
_____

But I have to say goodbye because...

_____
_____
_____

I've grown by...

_____
_____
_____

Goodbye,

_____

This is important for our healing because it allows us to dictate what we will allow from a person. It stops people from manipulating, violating, or using us. Boundaries can change from season to season or even person to person. Setting a boundary can look like, "Please do not call me after 9 p.m. on weekdays." Boundaries can also look like, "I'm not going to keep talking to you if you continue to talk to me in that manner."

Let's set boundaries and plan on sticking to them, for the sake of our healing journey.

Boundary 1:

_____

_____

_____

Why is setting this boundary important?

_____

_____

_____

Boundary 2:

_____

_____

_____

Why is setting this boundary important?

_____

_____

_____

Boundary 3:

_____

_____

_____

Why is setting this boundary important?

_____

_____

_____

Boundary 4:

_____

_____

_____

Why is setting this boundary important?

_____

_____

_____

Boundary 5:

_____

_____

_____

Why is setting this boundary important?

_____

_____

_____

Boundary 6:

_____

_____

_____

Why is setting this boundary important?

_____

_____

_____

FORGIVING AND FORGETTING

What emotion(s) did you feel when they wronged you?

_____

_____

_____

What would it take for you to forgive them?

_____

_____

_____

How is holding on to this affecting you and your life? Are you mentally sick? Physically sick? Does it feel heavy?

_____

_____

_____

What would you tell this person right now if they were in front of you? Be real and honest.

_____

_____

_____

I need to forgive because...

_____

_____

_____

I'm grateful for... _____

because _____

_____

_____

I know God is working on me because...

_____

_____

_____

Moving On

Once you truly forgive, it's easier for you to move on. I've had to forgive people in my life who have wronged me, abandoned me, or betrayed me. Sometimes it was a simple process, sometimes it took months or even years. Whatever the case may be, it can be done when you exert your energy into the act of recalling, forgiving, and moving on.

Holding on to the hurt and pain is only affecting you. Let go, so you can breathe again.

Here's a quick and simple breathing technique to calm yourself when you start to feel tense throughout the process.

4...7...8...

Do this sitting or standing.

Breathe in through your nose for 4 seconds.
Hold your breath for 7 seconds.
Exhale out of your mouth for 8 seconds.
Repeat until you feel the tension or anxiety ease up some.

Although this is the mental health portion of this chapter, let me just say, God forgives us every day for our transgressions. We mess up repeatedly. We should be more like Him, no matter how bad the hurt was.

EALA Prayer for Today

Dear God,

Thank You for... _____

_____

_____

_____

Please (ask for what you need and want)... _____

_____

_____

_____

I'm sorry for (confess and ask forgiveness)...

_____

_____

_____

Protect me from...

_____

_____

_____

In Jesus' name,

Amen

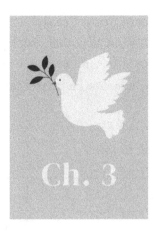

Ch. 3

Re-Newed

"Create in me a clean heart, O God;
and renew a right spirit within me."

(Psalm 51:10 KJV)

How this speaks to me:

Girl! When I used to hear this scripture, I didn't understand at first. As I have gotten older and have lived an imperfect life, I now understand. Oh, and how amazing it is to have this to be an option within my life.

As stated in the last chapter, "We live in a world where people and ourselves are our toughest critics, where God has already accepted our apology and made us white as snow."

Having a clean heart is having a heart free of pain, heartache, trouble, and even disobedience. Asking for a clean heart declares to the Lord that you are ready to walk with Him on a journey to peace, obedience, and righteousness.

Tip: Don't wait until you're "ready" (perfect); God accepts imperfection, hurt, pain, scars, all of that. Ask for a clean heart today; tomorrow is not promised for any man or woman. Start living for God now. Your journey may not be perfect but perfection isn't the goal; salvation is.

How does this speak to you?

_____

_____

_____

_____

_____

_____

_____

_____

_____

_____

_____

_____

_____

_____

_____

_____

_____

_____

_____

_____

_____

PRAYER

Heavenly Father, we come to You asking You to heal our minds and our spirits like only You can. We know in Your Word You said we would be healed if only we could touch the hem of Your garment, like the woman with the blood disorder. Lord, I know You can heal us too. Help us overcome every challenging period in our lives. We feel helpless and broken; give us the strength to carry on. In Jesus' name,

Amen

Re-Newed Spirit

So girl, look, to renew basically means to start again or resume. Often, this is what we have to do when we lose focus and fall off somewhat/backslide. What's important is you've noticed your downfall and want to restore your relationship with Jesus Christ. Just know He's ready when you are.

As stated previously, God isn't looking for a perfect version of yourself. God accepts broken, bruised, and imperfect people with the expectation you'll match the version in His plan one day. Girl, you are enough and if no one has ever told you that, please listen and hear God's voice declare it over you.

"Come as you are," my mama would tell you, isn't how you come to church dressed, it's how you come to the Lord with your heart, wherever you meet Him. your heart in the state it's currently in, being accepted and able to be wiped clean.

Renewing your spirit is easy. The decision may be tough, but the actual act of renewing your spirit, heart, mind, and soul can be a simple task.

1) Submit to Him (offer yourself back to Him)
2) Baptize to be washed clean
3) Live for Him
4) Pray always

Tip: Don't Wait!

Lord, give me discernment in all areas of my life, especially...

_____

_____

_____

How does "renew my mind with Your promises" speak to you?

_____

_____

_____

Lord, please renew my spirit in this specific area...

_____

_____

_____

This is important to me because...

_____

_____

_____

I know it can seem overwhelming, boring, and even uninteresting, but journaling is a major coping skill used to get it out of your head! Dump it all here. Lay your heart out; this journal is meant to be private unless you decide to share with your pastor and/ or therapist.

Take your time; don't rush.

JOURNAL PROMPTS

Choose from these to renew your spirit, or even create your own.

God is telling me to...
Why is it hard for me to apologize?
When do I feel the most distant from God?
What scripture shows me God's love and why?
What scripture brings me joy and why?
What idols in my life do I need to get rid of?
What is my spiritual life lacking?
What struggles do I want to overcome?
Reflect on scripture Romans 12:2.
Reflect on scripture 2 Corinthians 4:16.
Lord, in Your presence I...
A song that helps me feel closer to God is___ because...
To me, having the faith of a mustard seed means...

PROMPT SELECTED

_____

_____

_____

JOURNAL

_____

_____

_____

_____

_____

_____

_____

_____

_____

_____

_____

_____

_____

_____

_____

_____

_____

_____

PROMPT SELECTED

_____
_____
_____

JOURNAL

_____
_____
_____
_____
_____
_____
_____
_____
_____
_____
_____
_____
_____
_____
_____
_____
_____
_____
_____

PROMPT SELECTED

_____

_____

_____

JOURNAL

_____

_____

_____

_____

_____

_____

_____

_____

_____

_____

_____

_____

_____

_____

_____

_____

_____

_____

_____

_____

_____

PROMPT SELECTED

_____

_____

_____

JOURNAL

_____

_____

_____

_____

_____

_____

_____

_____

_____

_____

_____

_____

_____

_____

_____

_____

_____

_____

_____

_____

PROMPT SELECTED

_____

_____

_____

JOURNAL

_____

_____

_____

_____

_____

_____

_____

_____

_____

_____

_____

_____

_____

_____

_____

_____

_____

_____

_____

_____

_____

_____

_____

JOURNAL

_____

_____

_____

_____

_____

_____

_____

_____

_____

_____

_____

_____

_____

_____

_____

_____

_____

_____

_____

PROMPT SELECTED

_____

_____

_____

JOURNAL

_____

_____

_____

_____

_____

_____

_____

_____

_____

_____

_____

_____

_____

_____

_____

_____

_____

_____

_____

PROMPT SELECTED

_____

_____

_____

JOURNAL

_____

_____

_____

_____

_____

_____

_____

_____

_____

_____

_____

_____

_____

_____

_____

_____

_____

_____

_____

PROMPT SELECTED

_____

_____

_____

JOURNAL

_____

_____

_____

_____

_____

_____

_____

_____

_____

_____

_____

_____

_____

_____

_____

_____

_____

_____

_____

_____

_____

_____

_____

❧

JOURNAL

_____

_____

_____

_____

_____

_____

_____

_____

_____

_____

_____

_____

_____

_____

_____

_____

_____

_____

_____

_____

_____

"He'll restore all things lost."

Re-Newed Mind

Renewing your mind is similar to your spirit. It can be difficult to do, don't get me wrong, but it's possible.

Renewing your mind means changing your thought process and how to control it and what you allow in and out.

Renewing your mind is important, in my opinion, because it allows you to grow and change, and sometimes change is good.

When you renew your mind, it takes a lot of discipline but girl, you can do it! I have faith in you, even if no one else does.

UNLEARNING OLD HABITS

Why should you change? What is the benefit?

_____

_____

_____

What will you replace those habits with (positive)?

_____

_____

_____

How will you stay consistent?

_____

_____

_____

Who are you doing this for?

_____

_____

_____

Mindfulness Practice

Mindfulness is being aware of what is happening right now and accepting it for what it is. Focus on nothing else but your breaths and how your body feels in the moment. Use this exercise to help ground you. Look around the room you're in and find these 15 things. Use this practice wherever! 5...4...3...2...1...

5 Things you can see

1_____

2_____

3_____

4_____

5_____

4 Things you can hear

1_____

2_____

3_____

4_____

3 Things you can feel

1_____

2_____

3_____

2 Things you can smell

1_____

2_____

1 Thing you can taste

1_____

Version of Myself

Here you'll write down the rumors and the truths. Remember, there are three sides to every story: theirs, yours, and the truth. The hope is you'll discover who you really are.

How they see me:

_____

_____

_____

_____

How I see myself:

_____

_____

_____

_____

_____

The real me:

_____

_____

_____

_____

_____

If you met yourself, would you like you?

Yes or No

Why or Why Not?

When do you feel most like yourself?

_____
_____
_____

What do you like about yourself the most?

_____
_____
_____

How do you self-sabotage and how can you overcome it?

_____
_____
_____

"And God said, 'Let us make man in our image, after our likeness.'"
(Genesis 1:26 KJV)

Once you've renewed your mind, you will find it easier to be assertive and stand up for yourself. Use these tips in order to find and use your voice properly.

1) Gather your thoughts; pray about it. Don't act impulsively.
2) Be assertive, not aggressive or passive aggressive. This means knowing what you want and mean but being respectful yet firm.
3) Don't apologize! You feel how you feel; no need to apologize for it.
4) Be ready to compromise. Even though you have feelings, others do too. Meet somewhere in the middle with the outcome.

TAKING A BREAK

Sometimes we have to take a break. We have to listen to our bodies,. Girl, let's face it, sometimes we just need rest! Sometimes that can look like calling off from work and having a self-care/self-love day. Sometimes it can look like a counseling session, or sometimes it can look like taking a nice bubble bath after work and turning off your phone! Either way, you need it; it's important to let your mind rest sometimes. It's also important to treat your mind like you would the rest of your body if it were injured or strained. GIVE IT A BREAK! It's okay, I promise.

Some days will be easier than others; some days will be tougher than most. Make sure you speak up for yourself; be your own advocate. Only you know what you truly need.

"YOUR VOICE MATTERS!
IF YOU DON'T USE IT YOU'LL LOSE IT!"

CELEBRATING MY ACCOMPLISHMENTS

Write about one major accomplishment you've made within the past year. (What it was, how you accomplished it, who you did it for and why, and how you felt once you accomplished it.)

_____

_____

_____

_____

_____

_____

_____

_____

_____

_____

_____

_____

_____

_____

_____

_____

_____

_____

A Prayer for Today

Dear God,

Thank You for... _____
_____
_____

Please (ask for what you need and want)... _____
_____
_____
_____

I'm sorry for (confess and ask forgiveness)... _____
_____
_____
_____

Protect me from... _____
_____
_____
_____

In Jesus' name,

Amen

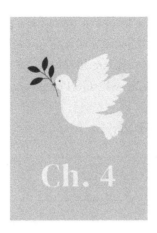

Ch. 4

Fearfully and Wonderfully Made

"I will praise thee; for I am fearfully and wonderfully made: marvelous are thy works; And that my soul knoweth right well."

(Psalm 139:14 KJV)

How this speaks to me:

Honey, let me tell you, if no one else has ever told you; you are fearfully and wonderfully made! What does that mean exactly? Well, to me, it means you are divine, you are someone made with a purpose in mind, not made of your parents' whole intent but of God's plan. You were designed with carefulness and precision with the purpose to help others be brought to Christ. What isn't fearful and wonderful about that?

I struggled with that for years with "I'm too big, I'm not smart enough, I have a mental illness."

I've learned that the level I'm on is for a purpose, and oh, how many people I've helped because of my "imperfections."

Tip: Don't let anyone discredit who God made you to be. Every "flaw" you see is a bonus to why God made you the way you are.

How does this speak to you?

_____

_____

_____

_____

_____

_____

_____

_____

_____

_____

_____

_____

_____

_____

_____

_____

_____

_____

_____

_____

_____

_____

_____

_____

_____

Prayer

Dear Lord in heaven,

I come to You today in order to ask You something simple: help this woman on her journey, help her to learn her worth and know and understand who she is through You. In Jesus's name,

Amen

Greater than Expected

By now we are friends, so let me say, sis, friend, you are greater than expected! There's no doubt in my mind on that one. I know this because you're doing this journal. It takes a great woman to want to better herself and her relationship with God.

So let's be honest with each other. Since we are friends, I also know you are greater than expected because of Who created you, Who formed you in your mother's womb; despite her issues or anyone else's issues, you were formed. That makes you greater than expected.

This, in fact, is the hardest chapter I wrote; it's also the last chapter I wrote.

Why?

Because this is something I struggle with today. Knowing that I am who God made me to be, on purpose. This is true from my mental illness to my size, skin color, and gender. It's hard being a woman who has a bipolar disorder, and along with all of this, happens to be black. People don't seem to have a lot of grace for people in any of those categories.

But it's important to focus on the grace God gives us, not the grace of man, because one is far greater. One created you in His image and one can't see past your "flaws" because they are different than theirs.

You were created to be different and to stand out in different and difficult ways. You were made to change nations, and no average Jane could do so. Your differences make you great. Your differences make you who God designed you to be.

In my trial sermon to become a minister, I preached about callings. In this sermon I mentioned that you can run from your calling but you can't hide. This also relates to who you are as a person. You can run from the person God created you to be, but you cannot hide from your true identity.

Tip: Be yourself, the person God created.

SPIRITUAL STRUGGLES

On a scale of 1-10, where is your spiritual life?

Low 1   2   3   4   5   6   7   8   9   10 High

How would you describe you in the spirit?

(I would describe myself as a woman who is growing into her faith. I would say I'm stronger now than ever but still have a lot of room to grow. Lastly, I would say I'm unashamed of my faith and most importantly my Creator, because without Him and the blood shed for me, I wouldn't be here).

_____
_____
_____
_____
_____
_____
_____
_____
_____
_____
_____

His Grace is Enough

{Free Kindness and Favor}

What is your greatest flaw (personally believed)?

_____

_____

_____

What is your biggest flaw (what they believe)?

_____

_____

_____

What qualities make you worthy of God's grace?

_____

_____

_____

What personal characteristics make you greater?

_____

_____

_____

Why should you have grace towards yourself?

_____

_____

_____

Bible Study

In Psalm 139:13-16 (MSG) it reads,

Oh yes, you shaped me first inside, then out; you formed me in
my mother's womb. I thank you, High God—you're breathtaking!
Body and soul, I am marvelously made! I worship in adoration—
what a creation! You know me inside and out, you know every bone
in my body; You know exactly how I was made, bit by bit, how I
was sculpted from nothing into something. Like an open book, you
watched me grow from conception to birth; all the stages of my life
were spread out before you, The days of my life all prepared before
I'd even lived one day.

What does this passage mean to you?

_____

_____

_____

_____

_____

_____

_____

_____

_____

_____

_____

_____

_____

_____

_____

_____

PRAY 'BOUT IT GIRL

To me it's so miraculous. First is the amazement I feel that the Lord selected me and formed me inside my mother's womb. How amazing it feels to be selected by the Most High to live life for Him. Next, because of the creation of my life and who made and designed me, that automatically makes me beautiful and marvelous, and nobody can change that; it is what it is. And nobody can change that for them either.

I'll forever worship and praise God just off those few facts stated above. He's so amazing and so precise. He's so precise that He knows us inside and out, every single thing about us. No doctor can compare. He doesn't have to use a CT machine; He already knows where everything is.

He knows how and why we were created and then born into the world, the stages which we'll go through and the reasons why. And lastly, all the days of our lives were carefully constructed before we have lived even one day.

Isn't that amazing, isn't that beyond what you or I could do? Isn't that what makes Him so omnipotent.

"The World Needs Who You Were Designed to Be."

Self-Love

You're perfect just the way you are. Of course, we still want to grow and become a better version of ourselves, but right now and forever, just know you are perfect the way you are.

You were made with special attention, flaws and all. In His eyes your flaws are perfection.

Loving yourself can be hard, especially in the world we live in. Girl, I know, what we see on Facebook and Instagram doesn't help us out at all. We must know in our hearts that we were created the way we are for a reason, and we don't need to change that, for anyone.

Loving yourself is important because if you don't do it, who else will (on the earth)? You have to set the example of what you will and will not allow in your life, in your personal space. You set the example by showing others how to love you. Not literally either, you just must love yourself. Get up girl, fix yourself up, and walk in a way to demonstrate it.

This means to take care of your personal hygiene, take care of your health (physical, spiritual, and mental), and walk in confidence.

Love yourself if no one else on this earth shows it; you deserve love even if it's just self-love. Show an appreciation for yourself.

What is Love?
You Are Worthy!

What does love mean to you?

_____

_____

_____

When is the last time you felt loved by yourself?

_____
_____
_____

How do you currently show yourself love?

_____
_____
_____

What is your love language? (circle one or two)

Words of Affirmation   Receiving Gifts
Physical Touch
Quality Time   Acts of Service
How will you use your love language for yourself?

_____
_____
_____

On this date _____ 20_____

I vow to love myself more, even in the simplest way.
Until we love ourselves first, we'll never love anyone else.
How are you feeling right now? What emotion?

_____
_____
_____

Are you being honest with yourself? How do you know?

_____

_____

_____

Are you in the present moment right now? If not, what is distracting you?

_____

_____

_____

How can you show yourself you love you more daily?
What would that feel and look like?

_____

_____

_____

Here are a few pages to write to yourself while you're on the journey to self-love. Here you can tell yourself why you're amazing and deserving of the love you give to others, and why you should give more to yourself.

_____

_____

_____

_____

_____

_____

_____

_____

_____

_____

_____

PRAY 'BOUT IT GIRL

A Prayer for Today

Dear God,

Thank You for...

_____

_____

_____

Please(ask for what you need and want)...

_____

_____

_____

I'm sorry for (confess and ask forgiveness)...

_____

_____

_____

Protect me from...

_____

_____

_____

In Jesus' name,

Amen

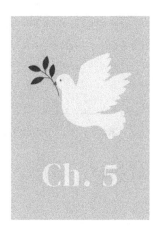

Recycle the Cycle

"Come unto me, all ye that labour and are heavy laden, and I will give you rest. Take my yoke upon you, and learn of me; for I am meek and lowly in heart; and ye shall find rest unto your souls. For my yoke is easy, and my burden is light."

(Mathew 11:28-30 KJV)

What this says to me:

There is a place where you can find peace and rest. You don't have to carry all your burdens alone, nor are you a burden. Rest in God's love for you. He'll never leave nor forsake you. Grace, peace, and salvation only come through God.

Lay down your burdens at His feet; have faith in Him, His sacrifice and blood. After doing this, you'll receive rest, a spiritual rest, a rest like no other, peace of mind and freedom within your soul.

I felt this recently, peace, and it was amazing. I felt peace after fully surrendering my life and will over to God. I instantly felt my worries fade, my anxiety dissipate, and my sadness turn into joy.

Tip: Say a prayer every morning asking for peace and protection. After a month, see how safe, loved, and peaceful you feel.

How does this speak to you?

_____

_____

_____

_____

_____

_____

_____

_____

_____

_____

_____

_____

_____

_____

_____

_____

_____

_____

_____

_____

_____

_____

_____

PRAYER

Lord, we come so humbly into Your presence, asking You to break the chains placed on us by those before us. We ask that You keep working on us and guide us in the way we should go to make the change out of generational curses. We have fought battles that were not ours for too long and it stops here, with us. We ask for Your continued grace and mercy in knowing that we are only human and with that comes mistakes, so we ask for grace just in case. Lastly, Lord, we ask for strength, strength for our bodies and strength for our minds. Walls are getting ready to crumble on our behalf and we'll need Your strength to get through the rubble. Lord, we thank You for all You're doing now and will do in the future. These things we ask in Jesus' name,

Amen

Breaking Chains

Chains that bind us have no true hold over us when we know and love the Lord, because there is power behind that name of Jesus! Hallelujah! Amen!

What is God teaching you through your journey through the Bible?

_____

_____

_____

_____

_____

_____

_____

_____

What is God teaching you through my journey through mental health?

_____

_____

_____

_____

_____

_____

_____

_____

_____

_____

_____

_____

"A woman who heals herself, heals every woman around her."

Just like it says, hurt people do in fact hurt people. And most of the time they don't even want to hurt you. It's just learned behavior and that disfunction to them seems "normal".

What has plagued you that WILL end with you (abusive relationships, lack of empathy, addiction, etc....)?

_____

_____

_____

Why is it important to you to break this chain? What will you and others gain?

_____

_____

_____

There is power in prayer. Write a prayer asking God to break your chains and free you from whatever binds you.

_____

_____

_____

_____

POWER IN THE NAME OF JESUS

There is absolutely power in the name of Jesus. He's there to help you, but He won't do it if you don't ask. He's not going to jump in on you and stop what you have going on; He wants you to want Him.

Sometimes we have to stop blaming the ones connected to us for the problems we face and realize that we are no better. When we blame them, we miss the opportunity to clean up the mess, bringing the issues at hand to God and working through them with Him.

Let's focus on us and let's be honest.

What is your ultimate issue, not the issues of others?

_____

_____

_____

How does this affect you day to day?

_____

_____

_____

What would you look like without this issue?

_____

_____

_____

How badly do you want that new life for yourself?

1   2   3   4   5   6   7   8   9   10

PRAYER FOR THE CHAINS TO FALL

Dear God,

I come to You as humbly as I know how, first giving thanks and honor to You. Without You I wouldn't be here or be able to live through the things I do. Lord, I am tired; the devil repeatedly makes attempts to take all the focus off of You and put it on to me and what I want and need in this earthly body. I'm asking You to free me of all chains that bind me. I'm declaring that Satan will lose his hold on me and everyone connected to me. I pray that blessings be poured into me, that failure is no longer an option, that peace be with me and no weapon formed against me will be able to prosper. I pay that generational curses end today and that it starts with me. I pray that sickness, addiction, pain, hurt, and mental illness all be removed from me, my family, and my friends. I pray for wealth to come into our family, in a way that can be used to honor You. Lord, I come to You today to ask for healing, for I know with You, the Omnipotent, anything is possible. And I know that faith without works is dead. I'm asking all of this so I can see You on the other side; this I'm asking in Your Son Jesus' name.

Amen

"Faith Makes Things Possible, Not Easy!"

Change and Growth

Changing and growing is a part of life, and so important to our development mentally and as a person overall. When we change, we show that we can adapt to situations foreign to us. When we grow, we also show we can adapt but also that we were willing to do so.

When I first got called to ministry, I was willing to change (slightly) but definitely not ready to grow. I was still out in the world, doing earthly things, unable to see what I was truly missing out on because I thought I was missing out on nothing when in the world. Like that was the place to be. Disobedient I was, and it showed. The Lord still blessed me and covered me (I thank my praying mama and grandparents for that) but He was displeased with me and my inability to see what change and growth would allow me.

If I had been obedient and changed and grew, I wouldn't be in so many binds that I'm in now, even though I'm saved and on the right path.

Changing means doing something a different way and growth is seeing something different and acting/reacting differently. I was unable to do either, because I was blinded by what looked like sold gold but was really plated (barely).

Girl, it's challenging, but the reward is so worth it. This goes for your personal life, relationships, and your spiritual walk.

When you're growing as a Christian woman, you may feel from time to time alone. Please understand that you're never truly alone, for you have the Lord on your side. But your mindset plays a big part in believing and understanding that.

What two personal areas of your life do you need to work on (negative self-talk, making excuses, or even being nicer, etc...)?

1)_____

2)_____

Growth is also knowing that you can do anything (with God on your side)!

What three things can you do, no doubt about it? (This could be past, present, or future.)

1) _____

2)_____

What's one thing you need to tell you, about you?

1)_____

What's on your mind right now?

What does living an intentional life mean to you?

What's draining your energy at this moment
and how do you refuel?

What's something you can do to challenge yourself and grow?

What dreams or thoughts have been repetitive?

What is being told to you?

What doubts about life do you currently have?
How can you change these?

What do you want to accomplish in the next 30 days?

When you feel alone, how do you feel?
How can this change in a positive way?

What does success look like to you?

What are some new habits you need to begin?

What are some old habits you need to get rid of?

Are you demonstrating the qualities you admire in others?

What can you de-clutter mentally, emotionally,
and physically to find more peace?

PRAY 'BOUT IT GIRL

PRAY 'BOUT IT GIRL

PRAY 'BOUT IT GIRL

Precontemplation- You have no plan to change.

Contemplation- You're aware of the problem but unsure if you'll take immediate action.

Preparation- You have intent to make change happen.

Action- You're in the act of making the change.

Maintenance- You've mastered the change and are maintaining it, working at it daily.

Relapse- or Backsliding

CHANGING FOR THE BETTER

Girl, let's face it, change can be scary. Change can be for the better or for the worse. Here, let's focus on the better.

The change(s) you want to make are:

_____

_____

_____

What changes do you need to make in order to achieve this?

_____

_____

_____

_____

What could possibly interfere with you changing?

_____

_____

_____

How will you know that your plan is working?

_____

_____

_____

How will this impact your life when achieved?

_____

_____

_____

A Prayer for Today

Dear God,

Thank You for...

_____

_____

_____

Please (ask for what you need and want)...

_____

_____

_____

I'm sorry for (confess and ask forgiveness)...

_____

_____

_____

Protect me from...

_____

_____

_____

In Jesus' name,

Amen

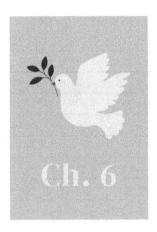

Ch. 6

The Best is Yet to Come

"Remember ye not the former things,
neither consider the things of old.
Behold, I will do a new thing;
now it shall spring forth;
shall ye not know it?

(Isaiah 43:18-19 KJV)

What this speaks to me:

To me this touches on the point of previous chapters (2 and 3); the past is the past, but also goes further in talking to us about not knowing what's to come to us in our future. God has promised us so much life and has given us so much hope. God's going to work a miracle, and we won't even know how it was possible.

Tip: Praise God in the good and bad times; don't forget to thank Him and give Him praise.

How does this speak to you?

_____
_____
_____
_____
_____
_____
_____
_____
_____
_____
_____
_____
_____
_____
_____
_____
_____
_____
_____
_____
_____
_____
_____
_____

PRAYER

Heavenly Father, we come before You to ask You to not only prepare a table for us in the presence of our enemies, but a table in a room full of greatness and excellence. We know that with You we cannot fail. We pray for greater in our lives in our singleness or marriages, in our careers and our callings. Lord, please prepare us for what's to come. We know all You do is great, so we expect nothing less than that. Lord, let us know that we are worth the wait. Let us see that we are worthy, and let us not get distracted by people or things. Let us be able to focus on You, Your direction, and Your voice. Fill our hearts to help us go in the way You want us to. Fill our lungs with air so we may send mighty praises up unto Thee. Fill our minds with Your Word so that we might be able to defend ourselves against evil. Help us to learn that we are as You say, these things we ask in Your Son Jesus' name,

Amen

Room for Greater

You're worth the wait of coming into your purpose.
I SAID, "You're worth the wait of coming into your purpose."

This journal is the perfect example. I became discouraged in the middle of creating it and I set it down for weeks. One cold wintery Sunday at church, I was reminded of my purpose and it was confirmed again later that same day, so I decided to pick the journal back up and complete it, this time with urgency.

I stopped working on it to begin with because of self-doubt and fear. As we know, those feelings are not of Him, so I had to send those thoughts to hell, back where they came from.

I'm actually writing this page with tears in my eyes because it's so fulfilling and I get such a warm feeling knowing that He thought of me when I was created and I'm able to live out His plan for me,. regardless of my past mistakes and failures.

PAUSES FOR PRAISE BREAK IN THE KITCHEN

The room I see and the room God created, even though the same room, my version isn't as clear as the Lord's. My version doesn't have much space and feels cramped and like a huge challenge and burden to face and fix. But I'm reminded that with God on my side, it's possible. His version is clear and He knows the outcome He desires. And that's it; my space does has room for greater, I just have to stop relying on myself to fill and fix it and make it right or it'll never get finished.

Tip: Please know and believe God is so good!

Fulfilling my Purpose

What's God's purpose for my life?

_____

_____

_____

Am I fulfilling my purpose?

Yes or No

What's holding me back?

_____

_____

_____

How do I need to change my outlook on fulfilling my purpose?

_____

_____

_____

What prayer can I say daily in order for God to reveal my purpose to me or help me fulfill it properly?

_____

_____

_____

Don't Get Distracted by People

Living in God's will won't be easy, and sometimes you may have to feel uncomfortable, but know God will NEVER leave your side. But we have to trust Him, trust that His plan is better than our vision.

This brings me to a time in my life where I was so confident in God. I felt so uplifted and invincible. I accepted my calling of being a minister, and I preached that first sermon, but just as quickly as I preached my first sermon, I ended up back in the world.

I was distracted by people, all the rumors, all the truths being flipped and twisted against me. But my biggest trigger was my grandma passing away. I lost faith, I lost hope.

People kept talking and whispering until I stopped and came out of my purpose. When I was drinking, they were quiet. When I was cursing and gossiping, they'd laugh with me. It's almost like I didn't matter anymore.

What does that mean? With God I was able to grab the attention of the devil, and all hell came out to stop me from reaching my full potential because the devil knows when I walk with the Lord and focus solely on Him, I can't be stopped. I'm that girl! So, whoever you are... Be that girl!

I AM

Who they think I am.

_____

_____

_____

_____

_____

_____

_____

_____

Who God says I am.

_____

_____

_____

_____

_____

_____

_____

_____

_____

_____

Tip: You are who God says you are. Your purpose has been predetermined, so there's nothing to it but doing it! God will protect you from the mess.

Staying on Task in my Purpose

Reminder: What is my purpose?

_____

_____

_____

What do I need to do to stay on task?

- _____
- _____
- _____
- _____
- _____
- _____

- _____
- _____
- _____
- _____
- _____
- _____

A prayer for increased focus and patience.

_____

_____

_____

_____

Sometimes we don't understand the path we're on, but He knows. Trusting in His plan and His direction is what faith is all about, believing in what we can't see.

> "Now faith is the substance of things hoped for,
> the evidence of things not seen."

(Hebrews 11:1 KJV)

Having faith is like "hoping" you'll make it from your driveway to the gas station when your gas light comes on before work, negating the part where you neglected to go to the gas station after work the previous night. "I'll go before work in the morning." Now you've woken up 45 minutes late, and there's no way you can squeeze getting gas into your schedule without being late. So now, you're hoping He'll make that insufficient gas in your tank sufficient enough to take you to work and to the gas station on your lunch break. You're hoping that a way will be made out of no way; that's faith.

Do you have faith in every possible and impossible situation though, or it is just the impossible moments? A possible moment can be made impossible in an instant; one wrong move from you or anyone involved can make that possible moment impossible.

You're at work and your computer crashes right before a raise-making presentation. Something you've prepared for for months, something that seemed like a given. You just told your best friend the night before, "Girl, I KNOW I'm getting a raise tomorrow; how could I not, I've prepared for this moment." Then boom! Something out of your control happens and makes the possible impossible. Now you're praying, right?

My question to you is, did you pray from the beginning? Even when it seems like it's in control, do you pray? Do you have more faith in Him than you have in yourself?

What's my point?

Sometimes we have more faith in our vision for our lives than we do in His plan for our lives, the reason we were created.

So my question to you...

Do you always have faith or just when it's convenient?

Do you have faith that the plans for you will not harm you or even make you unhappy in the end?

Do you have faith that, although scary, it's okay, knowing that the Lord will never leave you nor forsake you? (Hebrews 13:5 KJV)

Do you have even the smallest amount of faith, that of a mustard seed?

Do you have faith enough for the Lord to lead the way?

Do you pray, always?

The Lord wants to lead you to a place of righteousness. He will wait for you, but He can't do it for you. It must be a decision of your own free will.

Tip: Pray always, even when you feel like you don't need to, it's too simple of an ask. Remember to pray.

"God created you for a purpose."

Goals, Future, and Life Planning

Hey girl, I know, I know, planning for the future can be difficult, but it's necessary. This is especially true if you're really trying to "make moves" (achieve your goals). If not, you'll make decisions that are too fast and prejudged.

I'm a witness to this; I'm talking from experience. I was young (the common excuse) and I took out like twelve credit cards and maxed them all out. I'm talking all types of cards! With no way to pay each and every card on time each month; I mean, I was in college. Well, it's years later and now my life has had to adjust to unforeseen circumstances being a part of my life and unfortunately my credit score, BANKRUPTCY.

Girl, don't do it! That's the credit card part; never take out more than you can manage and never max them out. You'll pay for it later.

Planning for your future is so important. Having those goals in mind can help you when it comes to spending and making rash decisions. Learning about interest, loans, credit cards, bankruptcy, and even budgeting have mega benefits in a girl's life. This will help you reach your goals faster, without error.

TIP: Always think decisions over to make sure they are truly the best choice for you. Make sure you're not choosing a want over a need. Make sure you pray over big, life-changing decisions. Pray always.

My Goals

Here I'll write down my goals and check them off as achieved.

6 months

_____
_____
_____

1 year

_____
_____
_____

5 years

_____
_____
_____

15 years

_____
_____
_____

GOAL SETTING

6 month goal(s)

_____

_____

_____

Steps to achieving

1. _____

    _____

    _____

2. _____

    _____

    _____

3. _____

    _____

    _____

This goal is important to me because?

_____

_____

_____

What help/resources do I need to utilize?

_____

_____

_____

GOAL SETTING

1 year goal(s)

_____

_____

_____

Steps to achieving

1. _____

   _____

   _____

2. _____

   _____

   _____

3. _____

   _____

   _____

This goal is important to me because?

_____

_____

_____

What help/resources do I need to utilize?

_____

_____

_____

GOAL SETTING

5 year goal(s)

_____

_____

_____

Steps to achieving

1. _____

_____

_____

2. _____

_____

_____

3. _____

_____

_____

This goal is important to me because?

_____

_____

_____

What help/resources do I need to utilize?

_____

_____

_____

GOAL SETTING

15 year goal(s)

_____

_____

_____

Steps to achieving

1. _____

   _____

2. _____

   _____

3. _____

   _____

This goal is important to me because?

_____

_____

_____

What help/resources do I need to utilize?

_____

_____

_____

$ FINANCIAL PLANNING $

Monthly Income   Monthly Savings
$_____ $_____

Housing   Utilities
$_____ $_____

Debt   Groceries
$_____ $_____

Personal/Hygiene   Extras
$_____ $_____

$ Coming in $ Going out
$_____ $_____

Am I financially responsible?

Yes or No

Should I need to, how can I improve?

_____

_____

_____

$ FINANCIAL PLANNING $

Monthly Income

$_____

Monthly Savings

$_____

Housing

$_____

Utilities

$_____

Debt

$_____

Groceries

$_____

Personal/Hygiene

$_____

Extras

$_____

$ Coming in

$_____

$ Going out

$_____

Am I financially responsible?

Yes or No

Should I need to, how can I improve?

_____

_____

_____

$ Financial Planning $

Monthly Income

$_____

Monthly Savings

$_____

Housing

$_____

Utilities

$_____

Debt

$_____

Groceries

$_____

Personal/Hygiene

$_____

Extras

$_____

$ Coming in

$_____

$ Going out

$_____

Am I financially responsible?

Yes or No

Should I need to, how can I improve?

_____

_____

_____

$ Financial Planning $

Monthly Income

$_____

Monthly Savings

$_____

Housing

$_____

Utilities

$_____

Debt

$_____

Groceries

$_____

Personal/Hygiene

$_____

Extras

$_____

$ Coming in

$_____

$ Going out

$_____

Am I financially responsible?

Yes or No

Should I need to, how can I improve?

_____

_____

_____

$ FINANCIAL PLANNING $

Monthly Income

$_____

Monthly Savings

$_____

Housing

$_____

Utilities

$_____

Debt

$_____

Groceries

$_____

Personal/Hygiene

$_____

Extras

$_____

$ Coming in

$_____

$ Going out

$_____

Am I financially responsible?

Yes or No

Should I need to, how can I improve?

_____

_____

_____

$ FINANCIAL PLANNING $

Monthly Income

$_____

Monthly Savings

$_____

Housing

$_____

Utilities

$_____

Debt

$_____

Groceries

$_____

Personal/Hygiene

$_____

Extras

$_____

$ Coming in

$_____

$ Going out

$_____

Am I financially responsible?

Yes or No

Should I need to, how can I improve?

_____

_____

_____

A Prayer for Today

Dear God,

Thank You for...

_____
_____
_____

Please (ask for what you need and want)...

_____
_____
_____

I'm sorry for (confess and ask forgiveness)...

_____
_____
_____

Protect me from...

_____
_____
_____

In Jesus' name,

Amen

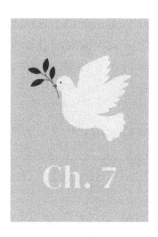

Be Still

"Be still, and know that I am God: I will be exalted among the heathen, I will be exalted in the earth."

(Psalm 46:10 KJV)

What this speaks to me:

Girlfriend, let me tell you, God IS who He says He is! Be not fearful or restless. Know that God has your back through it all. Worship Him and put Him first over anybody and everybody.

Quick story time: I've sinned, can you believe it? I've also doubted God in ways unimaginable. Even in those moments, long or short, I was still blessed day to day. If I wasn't, my life would have surely ended and I'd been cast away to the pits of hell. Even in those moments I was still told I have a purpose, even in my sin. But honey! When I tell you I acknowledged God as my Lord and Savior, and knew there was nothing or no one above Him, my life surely changed.

I didn't need drugs or alcohol to help "cure" the depression or loneliness, I didn't need instant gratification anymore, because the only one that could heal me was God.

Tip: Trust God first, understand and make Him your all in all, Alpha and Omega. When you believe that within your heart and soul, life changes and you can then share the goodness of God with others.

How does this speak to you?

_____

_____

_____

_____

_____

_____

_____

_____

_____

_____

_____

_____

_____

_____

_____

_____

_____

_____

_____

_____

_____

PRAYER

Dear Lord, help us to get to know You for who You are: awesome, omnipotent, the one true God. Help us to see that without You there is no other. Help us to understand that storms may come but You are able to calm such storms. Help us to understand and see that trials and tribulations we may face, but Your Word is true that patience within them shall get us through. Lord, we come to You asking to calm all anxious minds and hearts, to ease them into a peaceful place. We ask for depression to be gone from our minds and evil thoughts of harm to be banished. Lord, we need You now more than ever. Heal us, Lord, us women need to be healed. Help us to know that we are beautiful on the outside and help make us beautiful on the inside. Lord, these things we ask in Your Son Jesus' name.

Amen

During consecration New Year 2023, day two, my pastor said to the women, "When God fashioned you, He broke the mold. Your beauty transcends that of your physical appearance and radiates from within. Words cannot express how beautiful you are. Walk in that and rehearse this in your thoughts and mind. God has called you a beautiful creation. Who can disagree?" (2023, Jackson.)

It's true what he said; you are beautiful and it's not because of your outward appearance! You're beautiful because of your soul. You're beautiful because of how well you treat people and how you love others.

"He hath made every thing beautiful in his time:"

(Ecclesiastes 3:11 KJV)

Be Still and Know

"Be still and know" is actually one of my favorite scriptures in the Bible. Why? Because it is so true. Sometimes God is telling you to stop moving, not in a physical sense, but in a mental and spiritual sense. Are you listening to Him or is your mind filled with other things and desires? Are you really focused on Him or are you lukewarm in faith and action? Do you attend church faithfully and tithe when you go and when you're away? What does your prayer life look like? Most importantly, are you obedient?

In order to be obedient, you have to be still enough to listen and then act on His Word because you know His Word is what it is:; the most powerful.

How did I experience God throughout my day, week, or month?

_____

_____

_____

_____

_____

_____

_____

_____

_____

_____

_____

_____

_____

_____

Pray 'Bout It, Girl

The title of this journal comes from me, Jillian, losing faith in God and sinking down so deep. I would often hear a voice tell me to "pray." I'd politely ignore it and go about my business (not realizing my business is His). When I finally did begin to pray and regain my faith, stuff started happening. Walls started to tear down, and my life ultimately changed for the better, forever. Are you listening to God and His words being spoken over you? Are you talking back in prayer? Pray, always.

Prayer is so important because it's our chance for us to have a conversation with our Father. We can say whatever and won't be judged. We can also be forgiven and wiped clean.

"Girl" is being used in the slang tense, as in girlfriend, we are all friends here. As women we must learn to stick together and be nicer to one another, growing stronger with God, ourselves, and our sisters.

So, let's finish strong! You're almost to the finish line with this journal. But it's just the beginning of your relationship with God.

You've got this, girl, I just know you do! You've come this far, and I know you've changed so much already!

As my mama would say, "Keep pushing, you're not here for nothing."

BIBLE STUDY

Find a scripture about WAITING and write about it.

Scripture

_____

_____

_____

Breaking it down:

_____

_____

_____

_____

_____

_____

_____

_____

_____

_____

_____

_____

_____

_____

_____

_____

_____

_____

BIBLE STUDY

Find a scripture about WAITING and write about it.

Scripture

_____

_____

_____

Breaking it down:

_____

_____

_____

_____

_____

_____

_____

_____

_____

_____

_____

_____

_____

_____

_____

_____

_____

_____

BIBLE STUDY

Find a scripture about WAITING and write about it.

Scripture

_____
_____
_____

Breaking it down:

_____
_____
_____
_____
_____
_____
_____
_____
_____
_____
_____
_____
_____
_____
_____
_____
_____
_____
_____

BIBLE STUDY

Find a scripture about WAITING and write about it.

Scripture

_____

_____

_____

Breaking it down:

_____

_____

_____

_____

_____

_____

_____

_____

_____

_____

_____

_____

_____

_____

_____

_____

_____

_____

_____

_____

Find a scripture about WAITING and write about it.

Scripture

_____
_____
_____

Breaking it down:

_____
_____
_____
_____
_____
_____
_____
_____
_____
_____
_____
_____
_____
_____
_____
_____
_____

BIBLE STUDY

Find a scripture about WAITING and write about it.

Scripture

_____

_____

_____

Breaking it down:

_____

_____

_____

_____

_____

_____

_____

_____

_____

_____

_____

_____

_____

_____

_____

_____

_____

_____

_____

BIBLE STUDY

Find a scripture about WAITING and write about it.

Scripture

_____

_____

_____

Breaking it down:

_____

_____

_____

_____

_____

_____

_____

_____

_____

_____

_____

_____

_____

_____

_____

_____

_____

_____

_____

BIBLE STUDY

Find a scripture about WAITING and write about it.

Scripture

_____

_____

_____

Breaking it down:

_____

_____

_____

_____

_____

_____

_____

_____

_____

_____

_____

_____

_____

_____

_____

_____

_____

_____

_____

Bible Study

Find a scripture about WAITING and write about it.

Scripture

_____

_____

_____

Breaking it down:

_____

_____

_____

_____

_____

_____

_____

_____

_____

_____

_____

_____

_____

_____

_____

_____

_____

Find a scripture about WAITING and write about it.

Scripture

_____

_____

_____

Breaking it down:

_____

_____

_____

_____

_____

_____

_____

_____

_____

_____

_____

_____

_____

_____

_____

_____

_____

_____

Find a scripture about WAITING and write about it.

Scripture

_____
_____
_____

Breaking it down:

_____
_____
_____
_____
_____
_____
_____
_____
_____
_____
_____
_____
_____
_____
_____
_____
_____
_____
_____

"Cast ALL your anxiety on HIM because He cares for you."
1 Peter 5:7 NIV

Confidence

Confidence is something a lot of women lack because of what someone else has said. Today, we stop believing them and trust in what God has said about us and His Word, and how we truly feel about ourselves.

The work is hard and can open up some doors we've tried to shut, lock, and barricade. The result of building our confidence is beyond what we can imagine. It's getting places in life we couldn't before all because we lacked confidence.

> "In the fear of the LORD is strong confidence,"
> **(Proverbs 14:26 KJV)**

ALL ABOUT CONFIDENCE

3 things you like about yourself:

1. _____
2. _____
3. _____

3 challenges you've overcome:

1. _____
2. _____
3. _____

3 things you're grateful for:

1. _____
2. _____
3. _____

3 of the best compliments you've received:

1. _____
2. _____
3. _____

CONFIDENCE BUILDER

Think of 5 things YOU ARE and write them here.
I'll start you off.

1. _____I am blessed and highly favored!_____
2. _____
3. _____
4. _____
5. _____
6. _____

Now grab some sticky notes and put those
same things that you are around your house!

Confidence Affirmations

- I believe in myself and my abilities.
- I was created to do great things.
- Setbacks are not failures.
- I can challenge myself and not give up.
- 1)_____
- 2)_____
- 3) _____
- 4) _____

Confident Behaviors

1. Avoid negativity.
2. Use positive language.
3. Speak highly of yourself.
4. Say "No" when necessary.
5. Do everything with excellence.
6. Never feel "too good" to learn.
7. Set goals.
8. Set boundaries.
9. Be the example.

*You know who you are and are confident you'll live up to God's call for your life.

Week of:

_____

Monday- Today I accomplished:

_____

_____

Tuesday- I felt proud when:

_____

_____

Wednesday- Today was interesting because:

_____

_____

Thursday- I love myself more today because:

_____

_____

Friday- One person I helped was:

_____

_____

Saturday- One thing I did for myself was:

_____

_____

Sunday- A new thing I learned this week is:

_____

_____

Self-Esteem Journal

Week of:

_____

Monday- Today I accomplished:

_____

_____

Tuesday- I felt proud when:

_____

_____

Wednesday- Today was interesting because:

_____

_____

Thursday- I love myself more today because:

_____

_____

Friday- One person I helped was:

_____

_____

Saturday- One thing I did for myself was:

_____

_____

Sunday- A new thing I learned this week is:

_____

_____

SELF-ESTEEM JOURNAL

Week of:

_____

Monday- Today I accomplished:

_____

_____

Tuesday- I felt proud when:

_____

_____

Wednesday- Today was interesting because:

_____

_____

Thursday- I love myself more today because:

_____

_____

Friday- One person I helped was:

_____

_____

Saturday- One thing I did for myself was:

_____

_____

Sunday- A new thing I learned this week is:

_____

_____

Self-Esteem Journal
Week of:

_____

Monday- Today I accomplished:

_____

_____

Tuesday- I felt proud when:

_____

_____

Wednesday- Today was interesting because:

_____

_____

Thursday- I love myself more today because:

_____

_____

Friday- One person I helped was:

_____

_____

Saturday- One thing I did for myself was:

_____

_____

Sunday- A new thing I learned this week is:

_____

_____

SELF-ESTEEM JOURNAL

Week of:

_____

Monday- Today I accomplished:

_____

_____

Tuesday- I felt proud when:

_____

_____

Wednesday- Today was interesting because:

_____

_____

Thursday- I love myself more today because:

_____

_____

Friday- One person I helped was:

_____

_____

Saturday- One thing I did for myself was:

_____

_____

Sunday- A new thing I learned this week is:

_____

_____

SELF-ESTEEM JOURNAL

Week of:

_____

Monday- Today I accomplished:

_____

_____

Tuesday- I felt proud when:

_____

_____

Wednesday- Today was interesting because:

_____

_____

Thursday- I love myself more today because:

_____

_____

Friday- One person I helped was:

_____

_____

Saturday- One thing I did for myself was:

_____

_____

Sunday- A new thing I learned this week is:

_____

_____

SELF-ESTEEM JOURNAL

Week of:

_____

Monday- Today I accomplished:

_____

_____

Tuesday- I felt proud when:

_____

_____

Wednesday- Today was interesting because:

_____

_____

Thursday- I love myself more today because:

_____

_____

Friday- One person I helped was:

_____

_____

Saturday- One thing I did for myself was:

_____

_____

Sunday- A new thing I learned this week is:

_____

_____

A Prayer for Today

Dear God,

Thank you for...

_____
_____
_____

Please (ask for what you need and want)...

_____
_____
_____

I'm sorry for (confess and ask forgiveness)...

_____
_____
_____

Protect me from...

_____
_____
_____

In Jesus' name,

Amen

Tracking

Daily Prayers

Here you'll write out your daily prayers to God. It doesn't have to actually be daily, but when you feel the need, these pages are here.

Don't forget to add a different scripture each time so you can learn the Bible while you learn to pray. We pray when it's good and when it's bad. We pray ALWAYS. Lastly, don't forget to sign it with "in Your Son Jesus' name," just to make sure it gets to the right place!

Date _____

Bible Verse of the Day

_____
_____
_____

Dear God,

_____
_____
_____
_____
_____
_____
_____
_____
_____
_____
_____
_____
_____
_____
_____
_____
_____

Amen

DAILY PRAYERS

Date _____

Bible Verse of the Day

_____
_____
_____

Dear God,

_____
_____
_____
_____
_____
_____
_____
_____
_____
_____
_____
_____
_____
_____
_____
_____
_____

Amen

DAILY PRAYERS

Date _____

Bible Verse of the Day

_____
_____
_____

Dear God,

_____
_____
_____
_____
_____
_____
_____
_____
_____
_____
_____
_____
_____
_____
_____
_____
_____

Amen

Date _____

Bible Verse of the Day

_____

_____

_____

Dear God,

_____

_____

_____

_____

_____

_____

_____

_____

_____

_____

_____

_____

_____

_____

_____

_____

_____

Amen

Date _____

Bible Verse of the Day

_____

_____

_____

Dear God,

_____

_____

_____

_____

_____

_____

_____

_____

_____

_____

_____

_____

_____

_____

_____

Amen

Date _____

Bible Verse of the Day

_____
_____
_____

Dear God,

_____
_____
_____
_____
_____
_____
_____
_____
_____
_____
_____
_____
_____
_____
_____
_____

Amen

Date _____

Bible Verse of the Day

_____
_____
_____

Dear God,

_____
_____
_____
_____
_____
_____
_____
_____
_____
_____
_____
_____
_____
_____
_____
_____
_____

Amen

Date _____

Bible Verse of the Day

_____
_____
_____

Dear God,

_____
_____
_____
_____
_____
_____
_____
_____
_____
_____
_____
_____
_____
_____
_____

Amen

Date _____

Bible Verse of the Day

_____
_____
_____

Dear God,

_____
_____
_____
_____
_____
_____
_____
_____
_____
_____
_____
_____
_____
_____
_____
_____
_____

Amen

DAILY PRAYERS

Date _____

Bible Verse of the Day

_____
_____
_____

Dear God,

_____
_____
_____
_____
_____
_____
_____
_____
_____
_____
_____
_____
_____
_____
_____
_____
_____

Amen

Date _____

Bible Verse of the Day

_____
_____
_____

Dear God,

_____
_____
_____
_____
_____
_____
_____
_____
_____
_____
_____
_____
_____
_____
_____
_____

Amen

DAILY PRAYERS

Date _____

Bible Verse of the Day

_____
_____
_____

Dear God,

_____
_____
_____
_____
_____
_____
_____
_____
_____
_____
_____
_____
_____
_____
_____
_____
_____

Amen

DAILY PRAYERS

Date _____

Bible Verse of the Day

_____

_____

_____

Dear God,

_____

_____

_____

_____

_____

_____

_____

_____

_____

_____

_____

_____

_____

_____

_____

_____

_____

Amen

DAILY PRAYERS

Date _____

Bible Verse of the Day

_____
_____
_____

Dear God,

_____
_____
_____
_____
_____
_____
_____
_____
_____
_____
_____
_____
_____
_____
_____
_____
_____

Amen

Date _____

Bible Verse of the Day

_____
_____
_____

Dear God,

_____
_____
_____
_____
_____
_____
_____
_____
_____
_____
_____
_____
_____
_____
_____
_____

Amen

DAILY PRAYERS

Date _____

Bible Verse of the Day

_____
_____
_____

Dear God,

_____
_____
_____
_____
_____
_____
_____
_____
_____
_____
_____
_____
_____
_____
_____
_____
_____

Amen

DAILY PRAYERS

Date _____

Bible Verse of the Day

_____

_____

_____

Dear God,

_____

_____

_____

_____

_____

_____

_____

_____

_____

_____

_____

_____

_____

_____

_____

_____

_____

Amen

DAILY PRAYERS

Date _____

Bible Verse of the Day

_____
_____
_____

Dear God,

_____
_____
_____
_____
_____
_____
_____
_____
_____
_____
_____
_____
_____
_____
_____
_____

Amen

DAILY PRAYERS

Date _____

Bible Verse of the Day

_____
_____
_____

Dear God,

_____
_____
_____
_____
_____
_____
_____
_____
_____
_____
_____
_____
_____
_____
_____
_____
_____

Amen

Date _____

Bible Verse of the Day

_____

_____

_____

Dear God,

_____

_____

_____

_____

_____

_____

_____

_____

_____

_____

_____

_____

_____

_____

_____

_____

_____

Amen

DAILY PRAYERS

Date _____

Bible Verse of the Day

_____

_____

_____

Dear God,

_____

_____

_____

_____

_____

_____

_____

_____

_____

_____

_____

_____

_____

_____

_____

_____

_____

Amen

DAILY PRAYERS

Date _____

Bible Verse of the Day

_____
_____
_____

Dear God,

_____
_____
_____
_____
_____
_____
_____
_____
_____
_____
_____
_____
_____
_____
_____
_____

Amen

Date _____

Bible Verse of the Day

_____
_____
_____

Dear God,

_____
_____
_____
_____
_____
_____
_____
_____
_____
_____
_____
_____
_____
_____
_____
_____
_____

Amen

DAILY PRAYERS

Date _____

Bible Verse of the Day

_____
_____
_____

Dear God,

_____
_____
_____
_____
_____
_____
_____
_____
_____
_____
_____
_____
_____
_____
_____
_____

Amen

Date _____

Bible Verse of the Day

_____
_____
_____

Dear God,

_____
_____
_____
_____
_____
_____
_____
_____
_____
_____
_____
_____
_____
_____
_____
_____
_____

Amen

DAILY PRAYERS

Date _____

Bible Verse of the Day

_____

_____

_____

Dear God,

_____

_____

_____

_____

_____

_____

_____

_____

_____

_____

_____

_____

_____

_____

_____

_____

_____

Amen

DAILY PRAYERS

Date _____

Bible Verse of the Day

_____
_____
_____

Dear God,

_____
_____
_____
_____
_____
_____
_____
_____
_____
_____
_____
_____
_____
_____
_____
_____
_____

Amen

DAILY PRAYERS

Date _____

Bible Verse of the Day

_____
_____
_____

Dear God,

_____
_____
_____
_____
_____
_____
_____
_____
_____
_____
_____
_____
_____
_____
_____
_____
_____

Amen

Date _____

Bible Verse of the Day

_____

_____

_____

Dear God,

_____

_____

_____

_____

_____

_____

_____

_____

_____

_____

_____

_____

_____

_____

_____

_____

_____

Amen

DAILY PRAYERS

Date _____

Bile Verse of the Day

_____
_____
_____

Dear God,

_____
_____
_____
_____
_____
_____
_____
_____
_____
_____
_____
_____
_____
_____
_____
_____

Amen

Date _____

Bible Verse of the Day

_____

_____

_____

Dear God,

_____

_____

_____

_____

_____

_____

_____

_____

_____

_____

_____

_____

_____

_____

_____

_____

_____

Amen

Prayer Requests

When somebody asks you to pray for them, write it here. When you see someone struggling, write it here. Let us be all about intercessory prayers!

PRAYER REQUESTS

Who am I praying for?

_____

_____

_____

PRAYER

_____

_____

_____

_____

_____

_____

Who am I praying for?

_____

_____

_____

PRAYER

_____

_____

_____

_____

_____

_____

PRAY 'BOUT IT GIRL

PRAYER REQUESTS

Who am I praying for?

_____

_____

_____

PRAYER

_____

_____

_____

_____

_____

_____

Who am I praying for?

_____

_____

_____

PRAYER

_____

_____

_____

_____

_____

_____

Who am I praying for?

_____
_____
_____

PRAYER

_____
_____
_____
_____
_____
_____

Who am I praying for?

_____
_____
_____

PRAYER

_____
_____
_____
_____
_____
_____

PRAYER REQUESTS

Who am I praying for?

_____

_____

_____

PRAYER

_____

_____

_____

_____

_____

_____

Who am I praying for?

_____

_____

_____

PRAYER

_____

_____

_____

_____

_____

_____

Who am I praying for?

_____
_____
_____

PRAYER

_____
_____
_____
_____
_____
_____

Who am I praying for?

_____
_____
_____

PRAYER

_____
_____
_____
_____
_____
_____

PRAYER REQUESTS

Who am I praying for?

_____

_____

_____

PRAYER

_____

_____

_____

_____

_____

_____

Who am I praying for?

_____

_____

_____

PRAYER

_____

_____

_____

_____

_____

_____

Who am I praying for?

_____

_____

_____

PRAYER

_____

_____

_____

_____

_____

_____

Who am I praying for?

_____

_____

_____

PRAYER

_____

_____

_____

_____

_____

_____

Prayer Requests

Who am I praying for?

_____

_____

_____

PRAYER

_____

_____

_____

_____

_____

_____

Who am I praying for?

_____

_____

_____

PRAYER

_____

_____

_____

_____

_____

_____

Who am I praying for?

_____

_____

_____

PRAYER

_____

_____

_____

_____

_____

_____

Who am I praying for?

_____

_____

_____

PRAYER

_____

_____

_____

_____

_____

_____

Who am I praying for?

_____

_____

_____

PRAYER

_____

_____

_____

_____

_____

_____

Who am I praying for?

_____

_____

_____

PRAYER

_____

_____

_____

_____

_____

_____

Who am I praying for?

_____

_____

_____

PRAYER

_____

_____

_____

_____

_____

_____

Who am I praying for?

_____

_____

_____

PRAYER

_____

_____

_____

_____

_____

_____

210   PRAY 'BOUT IT GIRL

PRAYER REQUESTS

Who am I praying for?

_____
_____
_____

PRAYER

_____
_____
_____
_____
_____
_____

Who am I praying for?

_____
_____
_____

PRAYER

_____
_____
_____
_____
_____
_____

Who am I praying for?

_____
_____
_____

PRAYER

_____
_____
_____
_____
_____
_____

Who am I praying for?

_____
_____
_____

PRAYER

_____
_____
_____
_____
_____
_____

PRAYER REQUESTS

Who am I praying for?

_____

_____

_____

PRAYER

_____

_____

_____

_____

_____

_____

Who am I praying for?

_____

_____

_____

PRAYER

_____

_____

_____

_____

_____

_____

Who am I praying for?

_____

_____

_____

PRAYER

_____

_____

_____

_____

_____

_____

Who am I praying for?

_____

_____

_____

PRAYER

_____

_____

_____

_____

_____

_____

PRAYER REQUESTS

Who am I praying for?

_____

_____

_____

PRAYER

_____

_____

_____

_____

_____

_____

Who am I praying for?

_____

_____

_____

PRAYER

_____

_____

_____

_____

_____

_____

PRAYER REQUESTS

Who am I praying for?

_____
_____
_____

PRAYER

_____
_____
_____
_____
_____

Who am I praying for?

_____
_____
_____

PRAYER

_____
_____
_____
_____
_____

PRAY 'BOUT IT GIRL

PRAYER REQUESTS

Who am I praying for?

_____
_____
_____

PRAYER

_____
_____
_____
_____
_____
_____

Who am I praying for?

_____
_____
_____

PRAYER

_____
_____
_____
_____
_____
_____

Prayer Requests

Who am I praying for?

_____
_____
_____

PRAYER

_____
_____
_____
_____
_____
_____

Who am I praying for?

_____
_____
_____

PRAYER

_____
_____
_____
_____
_____
_____

PRAYER REQUESTS

Who am I praying for?

_____

_____

_____

PRAYER

_____

_____

_____

_____

_____

_____

Who am I praying for?

_____

_____

_____

PRAYER

_____

_____

_____

_____

_____

_____

Mood Tracker

Tracking your mood is important for mental health awareness. By the time you get to your doctor, you'll forget how you felt two weeks ago on Thursday. So track major emotional moments here. It's simple!

Mood Tracker

Our moods can change throughout the day. We could be upset and then pleasant, or we could be in a great mood all day. Let's track our moods; our moods can tell us a lot.

Date

_____

Previous Mood

_____

Current Mood

_____

How did I change or maintain my mood?

_____
_____
_____

What could I do differently next time?

_____
_____
_____

Pray for a better mood if your mood is low.

Pray for mood to maintain if your spirits are high.

MOOD TRACKER

Our moods can change throughout the day. We could be upset and then pleasant, or we could be in a great mood all day. Let's track our moods; our moods can tell us a lot.

Date

_____

Previous Mood

_____

Current Mood

_____

How did I change or maintain my mood?

_____
_____
_____

What could I do differently next time?

_____
_____
_____

Pray for a better mood if your mood is low.

Pray for mood to maintain if your spirits are high.

Mood Tracker

Our moods can change throughout the day. We could be upset and then pleasant, or we could be in a great mood all day. Let's track our moods; our moods can tell us a lot.

Date

_____

Previous Mood

_____

Current Mood

_____

How did I change or maintain my mood?

_____
_____
_____

What could I do differently next time?

_____
_____
_____

Pray for a better mood if your mood is low.

Pray for mood to maintain if your spirits are high.

MOOD TRACKER

Our moods can change throughout the day. We could be upset and then pleasant, or we could be in a great mood all day. Let's track our moods; our moods can tell us a lot.

Date

_____

Previous Mood

_____

Current Mood

_____

How did I change or maintain my mood?

_____
_____
_____

What could I do differently next time?

_____
_____
_____

Pray for a better mood if your mood is low.

Pray for mood to maintain if your spirits are high.

Mood Tracker

Our moods can change throughout the day. We could be upset and then pleasant, or we could be in a great mood all day. Let's track our moods; our moods can tell us a lot.

Date

_____

Previous Mood

_____

Current Mood

_____

How did I change or maintain my mood?

_____
_____
_____

What could I do differently next time?

_____
_____
_____

Pray for a better mood if your mood is low.

Pray for mood to maintain if your spirits are high.

Mood Tracker

Our moods can change throughout the day. We could be upset and then pleasant, or we could be in a great mood all day. Let's track our moods; our moods can tell us a lot.

Date

_____

Previous Mood

_____

Current Mood

_____

How did I change or maintain my mood?

_____

_____

_____

What could I do differently next time?

_____

_____

_____

Pray for a better mood if your mood is low.

Pray for mood to maintain if your spirits are high.

Mood Tracker

Our moods can change throughout the day. We could be upset and then pleasant, or we could be in a great mood all day. Let's track our moods; our moods can tell us a lot.

Date

_____

Previous Mood

_____

Current Mood

_____

How did I change or maintain my mood?

_____
_____
_____

What could I do differently next time?

_____
_____
_____

Pray for a better mood if your mood is low.

Pray for mood to maintain if your spirits are high.

MOOD TRACKER

Our moods can change throughout the day. We could be upset and then pleasant, or we could be in a great mood all day. Let's track our moods; our moods can tell us a lot.

Date

_____

Previous Mood

_____

Current Mood

_____

How did I change or maintain my mood?

_____

_____

_____

What could I do differently next time?

_____

_____

_____

Pray for a better mood if your mood is low.

Pray for mood to maintain if your spirits are high.

Mood Tracker

Our moods can change throughout the day. We could be upset and then pleasant, or we could be in a great mood all day. Let's track our moods; our moods can tell us a lot.

Date

_____

Previous Mood

_____

Current Mood

_____

How did I change or maintain my mood?

_____
_____
_____

What could I do differently next time?

_____
_____
_____

Pray for a better mood if your mood is low.

Pray for mood to maintain if your spirits are high.

MOOD TRACKER

Our moods can change throughout the day. We could be upset and then pleasant, or we could be in a great mood all day. Let's track our moods; our moods can tell us a lot.

Date

_____

Previous Mood

_____

Current Mood

_____

How did I change or maintain my mood?

_____

_____

_____

What could I do differently next time?

_____

_____

_____

Pray for a better mood if your mood is low.

Pray for mood to maintain if your spirits are high.

Mood Tracker

Our moods can change throughout the day. We could be upset and then pleasant, or we could be in a great mood all day. Let's track our moods; our moods can tell us a lot.

Date

_____

Previous Mood

_____

Current Mood

_____

How did I change or maintain my mood?

_____
_____
_____

What could I do differently next time?

_____
_____
_____

Pray for a better mood if your mood is low.

Pray for mood to maintain if your spirits are high.

MOOD TRACKER

Our moods can change throughout the day. We could be upset and then pleasant, or we could be in a great mood all day. Let's track our moods; our moods can tell us a lot.

Date

_____

Previous Mood

_____

Current Mood

_____

How did I change or maintain my mood?

_____
_____
_____

What could I do differently next time?

_____
_____
_____

Pray for a better mood if your mood is low.

Pray for mood to maintain if your spirits are high.

MOOD TRACKER

Our moods can change throughout the day. We could be upset and then pleasant, or we could be in a great mood all day. Let's track our moods; our moods can tell us a lot.

Date

_____

Previous Mood

_____

Current Mood

_____

How did I change or maintain my mood?

_____
_____
_____

What could I do differently next time?

_____
_____
_____

Pray for a better mood if your mood is low.

Pray for mood to maintain if your spirits are high.

Mood Tracker

Our moods can change throughout the day. We could be upset and then pleasant, or we could be in a great mood all day. Let's track our moods; our moods can tell us a lot.

Date

_____

Previous Mood

_____

Current Mood

_____

How did I change or maintain my mood?

_____

_____

_____

What could I do differently next time?

_____

_____

_____

Pray for a better mood if your mood is low.

Pray for mood to maintain if your spirits are high.

Mood Tracker

Our moods can change throughout the day. We could be upset and then pleasant, or we could be in a great mood all day. Let's track our moods; our moods can tell us a lot.

Date

_____

Previous Mood

_____

Current Mood

_____

How did I change or maintain my mood?

_____
_____
_____

What could I do differently next time?

_____
_____
_____

Pray for a better mood if your mood is low.

Pray for mood to maintain if your spirits are high.

"For as the body without the spirit is dead,
so faith without works is dead also."
(James 2:26 KJV)

Nothing is Impossible

Just as the title says, this is true. In this section you'll put all your desires, the prayer for that desire, the action(s) you'll take to achieve that desire, how you'll protect your mental health, and your faith decree (personal mantra).

Nothing it too hard or even too small for God to do for you. Nothing is impossible. Think of the impossible for you to accomplish, ask for Him to do it, put in the work behind it, and watch it be done. It won't look as tedious and challenging when you look back on it; watch!

Desired result

_____

_____

_____

Prayer

_____

_____

_____

Action you'll take

_____

_____

_____

How you'll protect your mental health

_____

_____

_____

Faith Decree

_____

_____

_____

Desired result

_____

_____

_____

Prayer

_____

_____

_____

Action you'll take

_____

_____

_____

How you'll protect your mental health

_____

_____

_____

Faith Decree

_____

_____

_____

Desired result

_____

_____

_____

Prayer

_____

_____

_____

Action you'll take

_____

_____

_____

How you'll protect your mental health

_____

_____

_____

Faith Decree

_____

_____

_____

Desired result

_____

_____

_____

Prayer

_____

_____

_____

Action you'll take

_____

_____

_____

How you'll protect your mental health

_____

_____

_____

Faith Decree

_____

_____

_____

Desired result

_____

_____

_____

Prayer

_____

_____

_____

Action you'll take

_____

_____

_____

How you'll protect your mental health

_____

_____

_____

Faith Decree

_____

_____

_____

Desired result

_____

_____

_____

Prayer

_____

_____

_____

Action you'll take

_____

_____

_____

How you'll protect your mental health

_____

_____

_____

Faith Decree

_____

_____

_____

Nothing is Impossible

Desired result

_____

_____

_____

Prayer

_____

_____

_____

Action you'll take

_____

_____

_____

How you'll protect your mental health

_____

_____

_____

Faith Decree

_____

_____

_____

NOTHING IS IMPOSSIBLE

Desired result

_____
_____
_____

Prayer

_____
_____
_____

Action you'll take

_____
_____
_____

How you'll protect your mental health

_____
_____
_____

Faith Decree

_____
_____
_____

Desired result

_____

_____

_____

Prayer

_____

_____

_____

Action you'll take

_____

_____

_____

How you'll protect your mental health

_____

_____

_____

Faith Decree

_____

_____

_____

NOTHING IS IMPOSSIBLE

Desired result

_____

_____

_____

Prayer

_____

_____

_____

Action you'll take

_____

_____

_____

How you'll protect your mental health

_____

_____

_____

Faith Decree

_____

_____

_____

Desired result

_____

_____

_____

Prayer

_____

_____

_____

Action you'll take

_____

_____

_____

How you'll protect your mental health

_____

_____

_____

Faith Decree

_____

_____

_____

Desired result

_____

_____

_____

Prayer

_____

_____

_____

Action you'll take

_____

_____

_____

How you'll protect your mental health

_____

_____

_____

Faith Decree

_____

_____

_____

Desired result

_____

_____

_____

Prayer

_____

_____

_____

Action you'll take

_____

_____

_____

How you'll protect your mental health

_____

_____

_____

Faith Decree

_____

_____

_____

NOTHING IS IMPOSSIBLE

Desired result

_____

_____

_____

Prayer

_____

_____

_____

Action you'll take

_____

_____

_____

How you'll protect your mental health

_____

_____

_____

Faith Decree

_____

_____

_____

Desired result

_____

_____

_____

Prayer

_____

_____

_____

Action you'll take

_____

_____

_____

How you'll protect your mental health

_____

_____

_____

Faith Decree

_____

_____

_____

NOTHING IS IMPOSSIBLE

Desired result

_____

_____

_____

Prayer

_____

_____

_____

Action you'll take

_____

_____

_____

How you'll protect your mental health

_____

_____

_____

Faith Decree

_____

_____

_____

Desired result

_____

_____

_____

Prayer

_____

_____

_____

Action you'll take

_____

_____

_____

How you'll protect your mental health

_____

_____

_____

Faith Decree

_____

_____

_____

NOTHING IS IMPOSSIBLE

Desired result

_____

_____

_____

Prayer

_____

_____

_____

Action you'll take

_____

_____

_____

How you'll protect your mental health

_____

_____

_____

Faith Decree

_____

_____

_____

Desired result

_____

_____

_____

Prayer

_____

_____

_____

Action you'll take

_____

_____

_____

How you'll protect your mental health

_____

_____

_____

Faith Decree

_____

_____

_____

Desired result

_____

_____

_____

Prayer

_____

_____

_____

Action you'll take

_____

_____

_____

How you'll protect your mental health

_____

_____

_____

Faith Decree

_____

_____

_____

Year Long Gratitude List

Here you'll write at least one thing you're grateful for each day.

1.
2.
3.
4.
5.
6.
7.
8.
9.
10.
11.
12.
13.
14.
15.
16.
17.
18.
19.
20.
21.
22.
23.
24.
25.
26.

Year Long Gratitude List

27.

28.

29.

30.

31.

32.

33.

34.

35.

36.

37.

38.

39.

40.

41.

42.

43.

44.

45.

46.

47.

48.

49.

50.

51.

52.

53.

54.

55.

Year Long Gratitude List

56.

57.

58.

59.

60.

61.

62.

63.

64.

65.

66.

67.

68.

69.

70.

71.

72.

73.

74.

75.

76.

77.

78.

79.

80.

81.

82.

83.

84.

Year Long Gratitude List

85.

86.

87.

88.

89.

90.

91.

92.

93.

94.

95.

96.

97.

98.

99.

100.

101.

102.

103.

104.

105.

106.

107.

108.

109.

110.

111.

112.

113.

Year Long Gratitude List

114.

115.

116.

117.

118.

119.

120.

121.

122.

123.

124.

125.

126.

127.

128.

129.

130.

131.

132.

133.

134.

135.

136.

137.

138.

139.

140.

141.

142.

143.
144.
145.
146.
147.
148.
149.
150.
151.
152.
153.
154.
155.
156.
157.
158.
159.
160.
161.
162.
163.
164.
165.
166.
167.
168.
169.
170.
171.

Year Long Gratitude List

172.

173.

174.

175.

176.

177.

178.

179.

180.

181.

182.

183.

184.

185.

186.

187.

188.

189.

190.

191.

192.

193.

194.

195.

196.

197.

198.

199.

200.

PRAY 'BOUT IT GIRL

Year Long Gratitude List

201.

202.

203.

204.

205.

206.

207.

208.

209.

210.

211.

212.

213.

214.

215.

216.

217.

218.

219.

220.

221.

222.

223.

224.

225.

226.

227.

228.

229.

Year Long Gratitude List

230.

231.

232.

233.

234.

235.

236.

237.

238.

239.

240.

241.

242.

243.

244.

245.

246.

247.

248.

249.

250.

251.

252.

253.

254.

255.

256.

257.

258.

259.

260.

261.

262.

263.

264.

265.

266.

267.

268.

269.

270.

271.

272.

273.

274.

275.

276.

277.

278.

279.

280.

281.

282.

283.

284.

285.

286.

287.

Year Long Gratitude List

288.

289.

290.

291.

292.

293.

294.

295.

296.

297.

298.

299.

300.

301.

302.

303.

304.

305.

306.

307.

308.

309.

310.

311.

312.

313.

314.

315.

316.

Year Long Gratitude List

317.

318.

319.

320.

321.

322.

323.

324.

325.

326.

327.

328.

329.

330.

331.

332.

333.

334.

335.

336.

337.

338.

339.

340.

341.

342.

343.

344.

345.

346.

347.

348.

349.

350.

351.

352.

353.

354.

355.

356.

357.

358.

359.

360.

361.

362.

363.

364.

365.

Additional Things to be Grateful For

_____
_____
_____
_____
_____
_____
_____
_____
_____
_____
_____
_____
_____
_____
_____
_____
_____
_____
_____
_____
_____
_____
_____
_____
_____
_____
_____

Graduation Ceremony

Congratulations, girl, you did it! I knew you could. Let me ask a couple more questions before you tuck this journal away and forget about it!

How do you feel spiritually?

_____
_____
_____

How do you feel mentally?

_____
_____
_____

What's your biggest takeaway?

_____
_____
_____

I'm so proud of you and hopefully you're proud of yourself too. I ask you to share this journal (not yours, a new one) with a girlfriend of yours to let her know how much you love her and the call you see over her life. I'm sure she's seen a change in you recently and is wondering how to go about it! Good luck on your never-ending walk with Jesus, and as always,

Pray 'Bout It, Girl!

Resource Page

Your Spiritual Resources

The Bible, Version Preferred _____

Pastor's Name _____

Pastor's Number ( )   -

Additional Support _____

Phone Number ( )   -

Your Local Mental Health Resources

Name_____

Phone Number ( )   -

Name_____

Phone Number ( )   -

Name_____

Phone Number ( )   -

Special shoutout/thank you to my Grandma Liz.
I hope you're looking down on me from heaven and are proud of me.
I know I'm doing things unimaginable.
Thank you for telling me to "pray always" and stay in my Word.
Thank you for placing your faith in me at a very young age and telling me I could accomplish anything I'd put my mind to as long as I had faith in Jesus.
Thank you for helping my mother raise me into the woman I am today.
Rules and ideas you had that I thought were silly really make sense now.
For your wisdom, I thank you.
Thank you for teaching me the Word of God.
Coming from a strong woman of God, and seeing your faith and strength through Him has made me that much stronger of a believer.
We both struggled in our own way and as you overcame, I shall too.
This too shall pass!
I'll love you forever.
Rest In Heavenly Peace, Grandma Elizabeth.

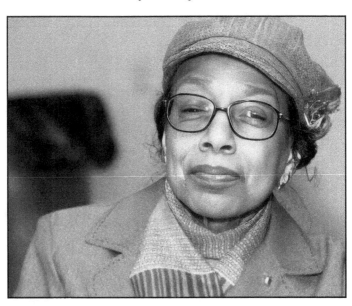

PRAY 'BOUT IT GIRL

(She Lived to Live Again)

A TIME FOR EVERYTHING

For everything there is a season,
a time for every activity under heaven.
A time to be born and a time to die.
A time to plant and a time to harvest.
A time to kill and a time to heal.
A time to tear down and a time to build up.
A time to cry and a time to laugh.
A time to grieve and a time to dance.
A time to scatter stones and a time to gather
stones.
A time to embrace and a time to turn away.
A time to search and a time to quit searching.
A time to keep and a time to throw away.
A time to tear and a time to mend.
A time to be quiet and a time to speak.
A time to love and a time to hate.
A time for war and a time for peace.

(Ecclesiastes 3:1-8 NLT)

Printed in the USA
CPSIA information can be obtained
at www.ICGtesting.com
LVHW011738070124
768357LV00001B/152

9 798890 416353